Melissa Panta

Aquatic physiotherapy intervention in chronic encephalopathy

Melissa Panta

Aquatic physiotherapy intervention in chronic encephalopathy

Case studies

ScienciaScripts

Imprint

Any brand names and product names mentioned in this book are subject to trademark, brand or patent protection and are trademarks or registered trademarks of their respective holders. The use of brand names, product names, common names, trade names, product descriptions etc. even without a particular marking in this work is in no way to be construed to mean that such names may be regarded as unrestricted in respect of trademark and brand protection legislation and could thus be used by anyone.

Cover image: www.ingimage.com

This book is a translation from the original published under ISBN 978-613-9-76238-5.

Publisher:
Sciencia Scripts
is a trademark of
Dodo Books Indian Ocean Ltd. and OmniScriptum S.R.L publishing group

120 High Road, East Finchley, London, N2 9ED, United Kingdom
Str. Armeneasca 28/1, office 1, Chisinau MD-2012, Republic of Moldova, Europe
Printed at: see last page
ISBN: 978-620-6-42251-8

ACKNOWLEDGEMENTS

We thank God for leading us here and forming this duo.

We thank UNASP for being an institution that has the best values and trains us to be excellent professionals.

We would like to thank our supervisor Abrahão for his support and guidance.

SUMMARY

Introduction: Chronic non-progressive encephalopathy (CNE), also known as cerebral palsy, is a disorder of movement and posture resulting from non-progressive damage to the immature or developing brain, which causes clinical manifestations (BAX et al., 2005). Physiotherapy treatment aims to minimise the consequences and promote maximum possible function, using techniques to reduce muscle hypertonia, minimise secondary problems such as shortening and contractures, increase range of movement, maximise selective motor control, muscle strength and motor coordination (BONOMO et al., 2007). Aquatic physiotherapy, indicated for the treatment of NPCS, is based on concepts of physiology and biomechanics. It utilises the physical properties of water (BONOMO, et al. 2007). The aim of this study was to analyse the effects of aquatic physiotherapy on patients with chronic non-progressive encephalopathy, with an emphasis on muscle strengthening; tone adjustment; postural balance; motor skills and respiratory function. Method: 16 articles were selected from the following databases: Medline, Lilacs, Scielo, PEDro, Crochane. Conclusion: Aquatic physiotherapy is a physiotherapeutic resource that contributes to the treatment of patients with NPCS, as it improves balance, motor coordination, temporal and spatial orientation, gait, muscle flexibility and social function. There is a need for studies with a larger number of homogeneous patients, control and experimental groups with statistical significance tests and treatments of choice for improving these aspects in these patients.

Key words: Cerebral palsy; Exercise therapy; Rehabilitation.

SUMMARY

CHAPTER 1

INTRODUCTION

Chronic non-progressive or non-evolving encephalopathy is a disorder of movement and posture resulting from non-progressive damage to the immature or developing brain (BAX et al., 2005).

Musculoskeletal and movement disorders are the main alterations secondary to brain injury (BAX et al., 2005; TRAHAN, MALOUIN, 2002; NAVARRO, et al., 2009).

The classification of chronic non-progressive encephalopathies of childhood is made taking into account the time of the lesion, the site of the lesion, the aetiology, symptomatology or topographical distribution. The most common form is spastic or pyramidal, which can manifest as monoplegia, hemiplegia, diplegia, triplegia or tetraplegia (ROTTA, 2002).

Physiotherapy treatment aims to minimise the consequences and promote maximum possible function, using techniques to reduce muscle hypertonia, minimise secondary problems such as shortening and contractures, increase range of movement, maximise selective motor control, muscle strength and motor coordination (BONOMO et al., 2007).

Hydrotherapy is an important physiotherapeutic resource that uses heated pools to treat a variety of dysfunctions (BARBOSA et al., 2006; HINMANN, HEYWOOD, 2007).

CHAPTER 2

METHODOLOGY

This is a bibliographic review of articles indexed in the Medline, SciELO, Lilacs, Pedro and COCHRANE databases from 2000 to 2016 in English, Portuguese and Spanish. The bibliographic search strategy used the descriptors "chronic non-progressive encephalopathy", "cerebral palsy" and "rehabilitation", and the combination with the descriptors "hydrotherapy", "hydrotherapy", with the refinement "aquatic physiotherapy", "aquatic therapy", "hydrokinesitherapy", "aquatic exercise", "aquatic activities", the search strategy used Boolean search logic, in which the keywords are linked with the connective "and", the selection was divided into two stages, reading the abstract of the articles and reading the articles in full, totalling 15 articles as described in figure 1.

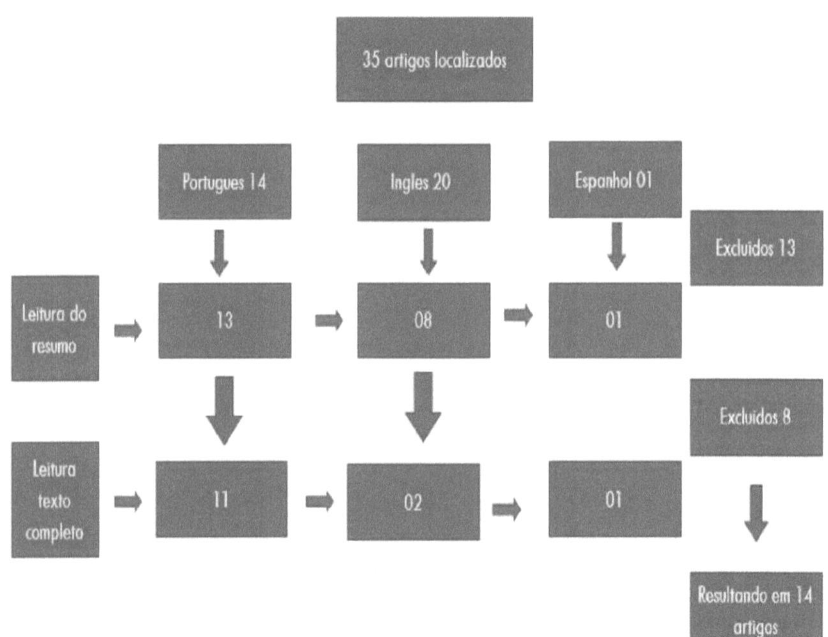

35 artigos localizados
Portugues 14
Ingles 20
Espanhol 01
Excluidos 13
Leitura do resumo
13
08
01
Leitura texto completo
11
02
01
Excluidos 8
Resultando em 14 artigos

Figure 1 -

CHAPTER 3

RESULT

Table 1.

AuthorYear of publication	CasuistlC af Age	Tip odc study	Evaluation method	OLjotlvo	Tim e Intervention	Result c conclusion
A1DAR *et al.* 2006.	N=27 children with CP 1.3 to 6.7 years$ Average 4.2 years.	Case series.	Technique; aquatic activities Tests; PEDI questionnaire part 1.	Evaluate the soci al function in patients undergoing an aquatic physical activity programme.	16 weeks, 2X7week for 3 weeks lasting 45 minutes.	Significant improvement p-id.05 at the social function level.
8ONOM0 er *st.* 2007.	N-7 cocb children Aged between 2 and 6 years. Average of 3.97 years and +V47.B4 months.	Unconfirmed clinical trial	Technique; hldroclnesiot orapia by melo from Bad Rngaz. Tests: Modified Ashworth Scale and PEDI parts 1, 2 and 3.	C heck functionality and tone.	20 sessions, 2X\week, 10 weeks lasting 40 mln.	Muscle tone unchanged. Improvement in PEDI skills in social interaction p<0.046, self-control p<D.O27 and mobility p"0.Q27.
TORRES et at. 2007.	N=22 children with CP, divided into an experiment al group with a mean age of 6.6 years, and a control group with a mean age of 3.7 years.	Study no experimental.	Technique; Bubatti on the ground and adapted in the water Tests: Modified Ashworth Scale and PEDI part 1.	Comparing two flsiotenapêuflco treatment methods; aquatic and conventional.	40 sessions; frequency c Intervention time not specified.	Both treatments were effective for children with spastic CP, improving spasticity.
ARROYOôf *ai.* 2007.	N=2 children with spastic CP, aged 7 (P2) and 12 (P1) years. Average 9 years ±3,63.	Descriptive and exploratory case studies.	Technique; hldroçlneslot ernpia through therapeutic exercise and manipulation technique. Tests: Adaptive psychomotor assessment; coordination	To investigate the influence of a programme of aquatic activities on the psychomotor behaviour of children with CP.	10 weeks, every week for 60 mln.	P1 improved 33% in coordination and balance, 14% in body schema, 40% in laterality, 17% in spatial orientation and 41% in temporal orientation. P2 improved 20 per cent in coordination and balance, 13 per cent in body schema, 28 per cent in laterality, 05 per cent in spatial orientation and 33

			assessment			per cent in temporal orientation.
			gorai, fine coordination and static and dynamic balance.			
ROSA *et al.* 2008	N" 1 10 years.	Descriptive study.	Technique: hydrokinesiotherapy through therapeutic exercise. Tostes: Manual of motor assessment and motor age.	To analyse motor development and the effects of a motor activity programme in the aquatic environment.	8 weeks, 2x/week for 45 min.	MI showed a 12-month increase in MI after the rehabilitation programme.
CHRYSAGIS *et al.* 2009.	N=6 13 to 20 years old. Average age 16. ±2.89.	Controlled clinical trial	Technique: swimming Tests: Scale of Motor Function Coarse, scale of	To check the effect of a swimming programme on the spasticity, motor function and ADM of undergraduate students.	10 weeks, 2x/week for 35 min.	There was a positive effect on motor activity, spasticity and ADM with a significant effect in relation to: active shoulder flexion (p = 0.052), active shoulder abduction (p = 0.052), abduction of the shoulder (p = 0.052).
			Ashworth, goniometry.	PC.		passive hip extension (p = 0.025) and passive knee extension (p = 0.045), interaction effect for spasticity of the hip adductors (p = 0.002) and knee flexors (p = 0.049).
PASTRELLO *et al.* 2009.	N=1 child aged 4 years and 4 months, with total CP.	Case study.	Technique: Watsu method. Tostes: Assessment of gross motor function (GMFM).	Verify the use of the Watsu method in aquatic physiotherapy process rehabilitation.	Stage 1. 16 sessions 30 min, 2x/ week for 8 weeks. Stage 2, 24 sessions for 30min . 2x\week for 8 weeks.	The Watsu method helps with motor rehabilitation and functionality by provide greater motor experiences.
ROCHA *et al.* 2009.	N=1 12-year-old child with CP.	Case study.	Technique: swimming. Tostes: physical and psychomotor activities	You will analyse contributions of swimming in the treatment of children with brain damage.	One year of observation.	Improved strength, balance. ADM, simple movements (joining hands).
ESPINDULA *et al.* 2010.	N=3 children with dlparetic CP, aged between 7 and 10 years. Average 8.5 years. ±1,6.	Case study.	Technique: hydrokinesiotherapy. Tests: Wells Flexometer.	Evaluate flexibility of the posterior muscle chain, before and after each hydrotherapy session.	4 weeks, 1x\week for 30 mln.	Hydrotherapy improves flexibility in relation to the posterior muscle chain, with an average gain of ±5.13cm.
LUCENA *et al.* 2012.	N=1 child aged 7 with CP	Case file.	Technique: hydrokinesiotherapy by therapeutic exercise. Tests Physiotherapy	Rolling over the case of a child with CP associated with intellectual disability, considering the	37 weeks. 2x a week for 40 to 60mln . This totalled 30 sessions on the ground and seven sessions	Improved postural adjustment and functional acidity.

			neurological assessment	importance of physiotherapy in the sequelae caused by this type of injury.	in the heated therapeutic pool.	
GETZ *et al.* 2012.	N-17 children with spastic diplegic CP,	Pilot study.	Technique: CPR stretching and Halliwick.	Evaluate metabolic expenditure in water and soil.	20 weeks. 2x\weeks for 30 mln.	The present study concluded that there was no significant difference in the re-evaluation of the PEDI and GMFM scales, but it was
POSSAMAI *etal.* 2013.	N=1 child aged 2 years and 6 months with spastic CP.	Case study.	Technique: kinesiotherapy Tests: PEDI and muscle tone assessment (Durlgon and Piemonte).	Checking for possible changes in muscle tone and fun ctional capacity CP patient, before and after aquatic physiotherapy intervention.	20 sessions, frequency and intervention time not specified...	De crease in spasticity and greater independence. There was no significant difference in functional capacity.
OLIVEIRA *et al.* - 2015.	N=6 children with spastic diparetic CP, aged between 5 and 8 years. Average 6.2 years *0.91.	Controlled clinical trial.	Technique: hydroki nesiotherapy by melode therapeutic exercise. Tests: BERG Functional Balance Scale; Dynanlc Galt Indx (DGI); Time Up and Go (TUG) Electromyography	Check aquatic physiotherapy balance children with PC.	16 sessions, twice a week for 35 minutes, for 8 weeks.	Improvement in BERG p<0.008; DGI p<0.005; TUG 01 p<0.022; 02 p<0.012; 03 p<0.007. in EMG there was an increase in muscle activation in the following areas transfers from sitting to standing and from standing to sitting and a reduction in standing posture without support.
POSSAMAI sf 17.2013.	N=1 child aged 2 years and ti months with spastic CP.	Case study.	Technique: UtCM kinesiotherapist. Toasts: PEDI s assessment of muscle tension {Durlgon and Piçmonle}.	Check for possible changes in muscle tone and in inte nded capacity CP patient before and after aquatic physiotherapy intervention.	20 sessions, frequency and time of Intervention not specified...	De crease in spasticity and greater independence. There was no significant difference in functional capacity.
OLIVEIRA oí */. - 2015.	N-â children with CP dlpatetlça .;H,:Ur . i. aged between 5 and 5. Average 6.2 snos *0.31.	Controlled clinical trial.	Technique; hldroclnosiot eraplap or melode therapeutic exercise. Tostes: Functional balance scale of BÉRG; Dynamlc Gqlt Indx ÍDGI); Time Up and Go (TUGJ Eletromiograf iade	Check aquatic physiotherapy balance childrenwm PC.	16 days a week for 35 minutes for 6 weeks.	Improvement in BERG p*0.006; OGI p<0.005; TUG 01 p<0.022; 02 p<Ú.O12; 03 p<0.007, in EMG there was an increase in muscle activation in the iransterance from sitting to standing and from standing to sitting and a decrease in standing posture without a pillow.
			(EMG).			

CHAPTER 4

DISCUSSION

The sample of the 15 articles consisted of 92 patients with ages ranging from 1 year to 34 years, with a mean age of 10.6 years.

AIDAR et al., 2006; BONOMO et al., 2007; TORRES et al 2007; GETZ *et al.*,2012; POSSAMAI et al., 2013; evaluated the PEDI, all use hydrokinesiotherapy as an intervention technique, TORRES et al., 2007; does not present statistically significant tests which prevents measuring this improvement, POSSAMAI et al., 2013 and GETZ et *al.*,2012; do not show a significant improvement, but AIDAR et al., 2006; BONOMO et al., 2007; show a statistically significant improvement as described in the previous table.

PASTRELLO *et al.*, 2009; LUCENA et al., 2012 evaluated motor skills and functional capacity respectively, using the Watsu Method and hydrokinesiotherapy, PASTRELLO *et al.,* 2009; reports that there was a significant difference but does not present evidence of this data, LUCENA et al., 2012, showed an improvement in 9 of the 18 requirements assessed, but without applying statistical significance tests, and it cannot be said that this improvement was due to hydrokinesiotherapy, since the hydrokinesiotherapy sessions were only 7 interventions compared to 30 physiotherapy sessions on the ground.

Table 2 - Summary of the articles' characteristics.

Author	What is the purpose of the study?	Type of ECNP/PC	What improvement	Objective achieved	p=O,Ú&	There was a worsening
Aldaret al 2006	Evaluating social function	Spastic and athetosis	Social function	8lm	p=0,05	No
Bonomo et al, 2007	Assess muscle tone and functionality	Spastic tetraparesis	Unaltered muscle tone, improved self-management skills, mobility and social function	SlrrVnfio	Social function p<0.046, self-confidence P<0.027 and mobility pcO.027.	No
Torres, ai ai, 2007	Comparing conventional and aquatic therapy	quadriparesis, cupiegia and hemiplegia, spastic	GMFM showed improvements in several aspects, with no difference between conventional and aquatic therapy	No	No	No
Chrysagis et al, 2000	Check for changes in tone, motor function and ADM with swimming	Tetraparesis and dIplegIa	Swimming had a positive effect on motor activity, spasticity and ADM	Yes	No	No
Pastrello et al, 2009	Verify the contribution of the Watsu method in rehabilitation	Tetra parebca	Improves functionality by promoting greater motor experiences	Yes	No	No
Rocha et al, 2009	Analysing the contributions of swimming	Ataxica	Improved strength, balance, ADM and simple movements	Yes	No	No
Splendula, et al, 2010	Wells and Dillom method in MMII posterior chain flexibility	Diparetic	Promotes relaxation, improves muscle tone when associated with passive stretching	Yes	No	No

	before and after hydrotherapy					
Lucena, "tal, 2012	Report on the case of a CP with an intellectual disability, taking into account the importance of physiotherapy	Diperotica	Mellvora of postural readjustment and functional capacity	Yes	**No**	No
Getz, et ei 2012	Evaluate metabolic expenditure in water and soil.	Spastic Diplogica	Patients had a higher metabolic expenditure in water than on the ground	Yes	**No**	No
Arroyo, et al 2007	Evaluating the influence of aquatic activity on psychomotor behaviour	Spastic	Improved coordination, balance, body schema, body orientation and laterality, spatial orientation.	Yes	**No**	No
Rosael al. 200B	Evaluating motor activities in the aquatic environment in motor development	**AtaxICa**	Motor age showed an increase of 12 months compared to Initial	**Yes**	No	**No**
Maciel et al, 2013	Identify changes in posture and balance	HemIpareOca	There was a global postural adjustment in those who underwent kinesiotherapy associated with hydrotherapy compared to those who did it only kinesiotherapy.	**SIrn**	No	No
Possamai, et al 2013	Checking home museum tone and functional capacity	Spastic	There was a reduction in spasticity, but no significant improvement in social capacity	Yes	No	NSo
Oliveira et al., 2015	Checking balance with aquatic physiotherapy intervention	Spastic Dysparesis	Improved speed and modified gait in certain tasks	Yes	Active shoulder flexion (p = 0.052), active shoulder abduction (p - 0.052), passive hip abduction (p = 0.025) and passive knee extension (p ■ 0.045), interaction effect for spasticity of the hip adductors (p = 0.002) and knee flexors (p = 0.045).	No

The articles selected analysed the topography of the patients, the presence of improvement, statistical significance (p<0.05) and possible worsening.

AIDAR et al., 2006; evaluated the social function of children with

CP, using aquatic exercises and a swimming programme that showed a significant improvement p<0.05 in the level of social function in the PEDI part1.

BONOMO et al., 2007; verified the hydrokinesiotherapeutic treatment in functionality and tone, which consists of Bad Ragaz, joint mobilisation, dissociation of waists and functional active mobilisation of trunk, upper limbs and hands, gait training with a 500g anklet and stretching. These patients underwent a pre- and post-intervention assessment, using the modified Ashworth Scale which showed no statistically significant change, PEDI parts 1, 2 and 3 in which there were changes in social function p<0.049, self-care p<0.027 and mobility p<0.027.

ARROYO et al., 2007; presented a study aimed at assessing the psychomotor behaviour of children with CP. An adapted psychomotor assessment of coordination, balance, body schema, laterality, spatial orientation and body orientation was carried out.

The patients were adapted to the aquatic environment, which consisted of breathing, floating, sliding, turning and propelling, starting the activities proposed by the assessors. Each activity was presented and carried out differently according to the results of the individual's assessment, with the focus being on the activities in which they showed the greatest deficit.

Playful activities were applied, music that varied in speed according to the exercise and intensity of the respective activities, stories and varied toys, floating materials, textures and sizes for proprioceptive and sensorimotor stimulation, as well as stimulation to favour displacement, imbalance, submersion activities were also presented, as well as on the surface and on the side edge of the pool, as well as activities to identify body parts. The results were presented separately for each individual P1: the patient showed an improvement of 33% compared to pre-rehabilitation in coordination and balance, 14% in body schema, 40% in laterality, 17% in spatial orientation and 41% in temporal orientation, there was also a gain in body muscle strength, as well as a significant improvement in his psychomotor aspect and improvement in muscle spasticity. P2: the patient showed an improvement of 21% compared to pre-rehabilitation in coordination and balance, 13% in body schema, 28% in laterality, 05% in spatial orientation and 33% in temporal orientation. The study shows that P2 had more movement experience than P1 as a result of having less motor impairment, as well as P2 showing less intense neural adaptation than P1. Aquatic activities are indicated for psychomotor stimulation of children with cerebral palsy and have a therapeutic effect.

TORRES et al., 2007 evaluated 2 groups of 11 individuals with spastic CP with topography of quadriparesis, diplegia and hemiplegia, using the modified Ashworth scale and GMFM as evaluation techniques, the 2 groups were divided into conventional therapy and aquatic therapy, each with 11 individuals, in conventional therapy the Bobath and Rood technique was used and in aquatic therapy the Bobath and Rood techniques adapted to the aquatic environment were used. There were two re-evaluations, one at the 20th session and the other at the 40th, where it was concluded that aquatic therapy cannot be recognised as the only influential factor in reducing muscle tone and that the GMFM showed improvement in several aspects.

ROSA et al., 2008; a study aimed to analyse the motor development of a 10-year-old child with ataxic cerebral palsy. The assessment consisted of the child's level of motor development using tasks that make up the Motor Assessment Manual, which analyses these items: fine and gross motor skills, balance, body schema, spatial organisation, temporal organisation and laterality.

The activities proposed were aimed at achieving autonomy in the aquatic environment, with the main focus on respiratory control and static and dynamic balance, movement in different positions and combining jumping with movement, activities such as walking, running, jumping, immersion, floating, sliding and movement in different positions and positions. At the end of the intervention, the same initial assessment was carried out, showing an improvement of 12 months in motor age.

CHRYSAGIS et al., 2009; verified the effect of a swimming programme on changes in tone, motor function and ADM in students with CP, using the modified Ashworth Scale, ADM with goniometry and GMFM gross motor function, dimensions D (standing) and E (walking, running and jumping) as evaluation methods.

 The swimming programme consisting of warm-up, backstroke, crawl, freestyle, stretching and relaxation had a positive effect on motor activity, spasticity and ROM, the swimming programme in the study indicates that an aquatic programme can have a positive effect on gross motor function, range of motion and spasticity, there was a positive effect on motor activity, spasticity and ROM with a significant effect in relation to: active shoulder flexion ($p = 0.052$), active shoulder abduction ($p = 0.052$), passive hip abduction ($p = 0.025$.) 001) and passive knee extension ($p = 0.045$), interaction effect for spasticity of the hip adductors ($p = 0.002$) and knee flexors ($p = 0.049$).

PASTRELLO et al., 2009, carried out an assessment using the Gross Motor Function Measure (GMFM) scale and measured gross motor assessment in dimensions A (lying and rolling) and B (sitting) with the GMFM scale. The study was divided into stages: Stage 1, 16 sessions for 30 minutes twice a week for 8 weeks, conventional therapy based on stimulation of the stages of typical neuro-psychomotor development, orthopaedic propaedeutics and manoeuvres on the Swiss ball. Stage 2, 24 sessions of 30 minutes twice a week for 8 weeks, with the same ground behaviour as stage 1, combined with the Watsu method in an indoor pool heated to 33° C. No floats, toys or other materials were used during the intervention.

According to the initial assessment, the following manoeuvres were established: breathing dance, offer, normal accordion, rotating accordion, spine rotation and hip swing, inside leg rotation, outside leg rotation, pendulum, monkey, knee to chest and ending with the hand on the heart's master point. This study showed no statistically significant increase in relation to the performance of assessments 1 and 2 in dimension A and no significant difference between the end of stage 1 and 2 in dimension B (p=0.05).

ROCHA et al., 2009; a case study with the aim of analysing the contributions of swimming in the treatment of children with CP. Physical and psychomotor activities were carried out in an aquatic environment over a period of one year, providing recreational activities, muscle strengthening, improved posture and range of movement.

The study concludes that swimming helps reduce muscle stiffness, increases range of motion, improves balance and muscle strength.

The study is not well evaluated using reliable evaluation methods, nor does it have a proven scientific basis, nor does it have quantitative scales to define the improvements presented.

ESPINDULA et al., 2010 used the Wells flexometer to measure the flexibility of the posterior muscle chain of children with CP after each hydrotherapy session, which consisted of stretching the triceps sural, hamstring, quadriceps and ankle mobilisation muscles, as well as stretching the flexor muscles of the upper limbs, in a series of four repetitions for 30 seconds of maintenance, totalling 30 minutes of intervention, showing a significant improvement in flexibility with an overall average of ± 5.13 cm.

GETZ el al., 2012, assessed two groups divided into an aquatic intervention group (9) and a ground intervention group (8), using the GMFM scale, PEDI, 10-metre walk test and metabolic measurement using the Cosmed K4B2 as assessment methods.

 Each child was assigned to an instructor, and the objectives of the activities were pre-established according to the results of each participant's individual assessment. The aquatic intervention was carried out twice a week for 30 minutes, consisting of 5 minutes of group activity, 20 minutes of individual activities using the Halliwick method and a final 5 minutes of relaxation with children's music.

The solo intervention lasted 15 to 20 minutes on a treadmill at a comfortable individualised speed, ranging from 0.5 to 1.0 km/h, and stretching. The present study concluded that there was no significant difference in the re-evaluation of the PEDI and GMFM scales, but greater metabolic expenditure was observed in individuals who underwent aquatic activity.

LUCENA et al.,2012 carried out a neurological assessment with a patient with spastic diplegic CP to check muscle tone. The therapeutic approach consisted of the Bobath method, stretching, hydrokinesiotherapy aimed at relieving muscle spasms, maintaining and/or increasing range of movement, strengthening muscles, improving blood circulation, improving motor coordination, balance and proprioception.

The article shows great improvements after two neurological assessments of children's motor development, but it doesn't present statistically significant data, and it can't be said that the improvement was due to hydrokinesiotherapy because there were 30 sessions on the ground and 7 in the aquatic environment.

OLIVEIRA et al., 2015, verified the interference of aquatic physiotherapy on the balance of children with CP, applying the BERG Functional Balance Scale; Dynamic Gait Indx (DGI); Time Up and Go (TUG) and Surface Electromyography (EMG), a protocol was carried out consisting of: trunk flexion with manual resistance, static and dynamic balance training, resisted dorsiflexion, weight unloading, gait training. There was a statistically significant improvement in BERG $p<0.008$; DGI $p<0.005$; TUG 01 $p<0.022$; 02 $p<0.012$; 03 $p<0.007$, in EMG there was an increase in muscle activation in transfers from sitting to standing and from standing to sitting and a decrease in standing posture without support.

CHAPTER 5

FINAL CONSIDERATION

Aquatic physiotherapy is a physiotherapeutic resource that contributes to the treatment of patients with NPCS, as it improves balance, motor coordination, temporal and spatial orientation, gait, muscle flexibility and social function. There is a need for studies with a larger number of homogeneous patients, control and experimental groups with statistical significance tests and treatments of choice for improving these aspects in these patients.

CHAPTER 6

BIBLIOGRAPHICAL REFERENCES

AIDAR, F. J.; CARNEIRO, A; SILVA, A.; REIS, V.; GARRIDO, N.; VIEIRA, R. cerebral palsy and aquatic activities: aspects related to health and social function. MOTRICIDADE v.2 n.2 p.109-116. 2006.

ARROYO, C. T.; OLIVEIRA, S. R. G.; AQUATIC ACTIVITY AND THE PSYCHOMOTRICITY OF CHILDREN WITH CEREBRAL PALSY. MOTRIZ. v.13 n.2 p.97-105. 2007.

BAX M, GOLDESTEIN M, ROSENBAUM P, PANETH N. Proposed definition and classification of cerebral palsy. Dev. Med Child Neurol. 2005; 47:571-76.

BONOMO, L. M. M; CASTRO, V. C; FERREIRA, D. M; MIYAMOTO, S. T. Hidroterapia na aquisição da funcionalidade de crianças com Paralisia Cerebral. Revista Neurociência. 2007; 15 (2):125-130.

CALCAGNO, N. C.; PINTO, T. P. S.; VAZ, D. V.; SAMPAIO, R. F. Analysing the effects of serial splinting in children with cerebral palsy: a systematic literature review. Rev. Bras. Saúde Matern. Infant. 2006; 6 (1): 11-22.

CARREGARO RL, TOLEDO AM. Physiological effects and scientific evidence of the effectiveness of aquatic physiotherapy. Revista Movimenta 2008; 1(1):23-7.

CHRYSAGIS, N.; DOUKA, A.; NIKOPOULOS, M.;

APOSTOLOPOULOU,F.; KOUTSOUKI,D. effects of an aquatic programme on gross motor function of children with spastic cerebral palsy. JBE. v.5 n.2 2009.

DIAMENT A. Chronic encephalopathy in childhood (cerebral palsy). In: DIAMENT A & CYPE A. editors. Child neurology. 3 ed. São Paulo: Atheneu, 1996. P.781-98.

ESPINDULA, A. P.; JAMMAL, M.P.; GUIMARAES, C.S.O.; ABATE, D. T. R. S.; REIS, M.A.; TEIXEIRA, V.P.A. evaluation of flexibility by the wells flexometer method in children with cerebral palsy submitted to hydrotherapeutic treatment: case study. ACTA. SCIENTIARUM. HEALTH SCIENCES. v.32 n.2 P.163-167. 2010.

GRETZ, M.; HUTZLER, Y., VERMEER, A.; YAROM, Y.;UNNITHAN,V. THE effect of aquatic and land-based training on the metabolic cost of walking and motor performance in children with cerebral palsy. ISRN Rehabilitation p.1-8 2012.

HINMANN RS, HEYWOOD SE, DAY AR. Aquatic Physical Therapy for Hip and Knee Osteoarthritis: Results of a Single-Blind Randomised Controlled Trial. Phys Ther. 2007;87(1):32-43.

JACQUES K. et al. Efficacy of hydrotherapy in children with non-progressive diachronic encephalopathy of childhood: a systematic review. Mov. , Curitiba, 2010; 23 (1):53-61.

LOW JA, GALBRAITH RS, MUIR DW, KILLEN HL, PATER EA, - KARCHMAR EJ. Mortality and mobidadity after intrapartum asphyxabin the preterm foetus. Obstet Gynecol 1992; 80(1):57-61.

LUCENA, M.O.V.; CARVALHO, S.M.C.R; GERMANO, C.D.F.M.; LEMOS, M.T.M. abordagem fisioterapeutica na visão do "cuidar" de uma criança com paralisia cerebral associada a deficiencia intelectual: relato de caso. Rev. Bras Ci Saude v.16 n.4 p.567-572. 2013.

MACIEL, F. ; MAZZITELLI, C. ; SÁ, C.S.C. posture and balance in children with cerebral palsy submitted to different therapeutic approaches. Rev. NEUROCIENC. V.21 n. 1 p.14 - 21. 2013

OLIVEIRA , L. M. M. ; BRAGA, D. M ; OLIVEIRA, L. C ; ALVES, T. L ; CYRILLO, F. N. ; KANASHIRO, M.S. interferência da fisioterapia aquática no equilíbrio de crianças com paralisia cerebral. rev. pesquisa em fisioterapia v.5 n.2 p. 70-82. 2015.

PASTRELLO, F. H. H.; GARÇAO, D. C.; PEREIRA, K. The watsu method as a complementary resource in the physiotherapy treatment of a child with spastic tetraparetic cerebral palsy: a case study. Fisioterapia Mov. v.22 n.1 p.95-102. 2009.

PATIKAS D, WOLF SI, ARMBRUST P, MUND K, SCHUSTER W, DREHER T, et al. Effects of a postoperative resistive exercise programme on the knee extension and flexion torque in children with cerebral palsy: a randomized clinical trial. Arch Phys Med Rehabil 2006; 87(9):1161- 1169.

POSSAMAI; M. F.; SANTOS, R. V. Aquatic physiotherapy in functionality and tonic modulation in patients with spastic cerebral palsy. Digital Magazine. V.18 n.187, 2013.

ROBERTSON C, SAUVE RS, CHRISTIANSON HE. Province-based study of neurologic disability among survivors weighing 500 through 1249 grams at birth. Paediatrics. 1994; 93:636-40.

ROSA, G. K. B.; MARQUES, I.; PAPST, J. M.; GOBBI, L. T. B. Motor development of children with cerebral palsy: evaluation and intervention. Revista Brasileira. v.14 n.2 p.163-176, 2008.

ROTHSTEIN JR, BELTRAME TS. Motor and biopsychosocial characteristics of children with cerebral palsy; Rev. Bras. Ci. e Mov. 2013; 21(3): 118-126.

ROTTA NT. Chronic childhood encephalopathy or cerebral palsy. In: Porto CC. Medical Semiology. 4 ed. Rio de Janeiro: Guanabara Koogan; 2001. P.1276-8.

ROTTA NT. Cerebral palsy, new therapeutic perspectives. J Pediatr. 2002; 78 (supl.1): S48-S53.

TORRES CP, VAN DEN BERG B, OECHSLI FW, CUMMINS S. Prenatal and perinatal factors in the etiology of cerebral palsy. J Paediatr 1990; 116(4):615-9.

TORRES, Y.; CASTILLO, A.; DIAZ, C. Evaluacion de um

programa de fisioterapia convencional más terapia acuática in minos com pardises cerebral espástica. Colomb. Rehabl. v.6 n.6 p.21-37, 2007.

TOVIN BJ, WOLF SL, GREENFIELD BH, CROUSE J, WOODFIN BA. Comparison of the effects of exercise in water and on land on the rehabilitation of patients with intra-articular anterior cruciate ligament reconstructions. Phis Ther. 1994;74(8):710-19.

TRAHAN J, MALOUIN F. Intermittent intensive physiotherapy in children with cerebral palsy: a pilot study. Dev Med Child Neurol. 2002;44:233-9.